ALEXANDER GRANT

Unshackling Anxiety: Empowering Strategies for Lasting Freedom

Disclaimer:

This book, titled "Unshackling Anxiety: Empowering Strategies for Lasting Freedom," is provided for informational purposes only and does not constitute medical advice. The author, although well-researched and experienced, is not a medical professional. The content of this book is based on personal research, life experiences, and general knowledge about anxiety. Readers should consult with qualified healthcare professionals for personalized advice and guidance regarding their specific anxiety concerns. The author and publisher cannot be held responsible for any actions taken based on the information provided in this book. Readers are responsible for their own choices and should exercise caution and discretion when implementing strategies or techniques mentioned.

Limitation of Liability:

The author and publisher of "Unshackling Anxiety: Empowering Strategies for Lasting Freedom" shall not be held liable for any direct, indirect, incidental, consequential, or special damages arising from the use or inability to use the information provided in this book. The information is provided on an "as-is" basis and is not intended to replace professional medical advice or treatment. Readers should seek appropriate professional help for their specific circumstances. The author and publisher do not warrant the accuracy, completeness, or timeliness of the information contained in this book. Any reliance on the information is at the reader's own risk. The author and publisher disclaim any and all liability for any damages or injuries, including but not limited to those caused by negligence or any failure of performance, error, omission, interruption, deletion, defect, delay in operation or transmission, computer virus, communication line failure, theft, or destruction.

First edition

ISBN: 9798852333551

Agent: Shazum Sheraz

This book was professionally typeset on Reedsy.
Find out more at reedsy.com

To Shaz,
Thank you for your unwavering support and inspiration.
This book is for you.

Alexander Grant

Contents

I

Understanding Anxiety

1

Introduction

Welcome to "Unshackling Anxiety: Empowering Strategies for Lasting Freedom." In this book, we embark on a transformative journey together—a journey aimed at unraveling the complexities of anxiety and equipping you with empowering strategies to overcome its grip. While I am not a medical professional, I share this book as a fellow traveler who has experienced anxiety firsthand and found ways to navigate its challenges.

Anxiety affects millions of people worldwide, casting a shadow over their lives and preventing them from fully embracing their true potential. It manifests in different forms—ranging from everyday worries to panic attacks—and can impact our mental, emotional, and physical well-being. However, it's important to remember that anxiety doesn't define you. You have the power within you to regain control and experience lasting freedom.

In this chapter, we'll set the stage by exploring the nature of anxiety and its far-reaching effects. By understanding anxiety at its core, we can begin to demystify its hold on our lives and work towards breaking free. Let's delve into the foundation upon which we'll build our empowering strategies.

In Chapter 1: Introduction, we will cover the following topics:

1. Defining Anxiety:We'll examine what anxiety truly means and explore its various manifestations. By gaining a deeper understanding of anxiety, we can begin to recognize its presence in our lives and develop a clearer perspective.

2. Exploring the Causes of Anxiety: Anxiety can have numerous triggers, ranging from external circumstances to internal factors. We'll delve into these potential causes and shed light on how they contribute to our experience of anxiety.

3. The Impact of Anxiety on Daily Life: Anxiety permeates various aspects of our existence, affecting our relationships, work, and overall well-being. We'll explore the far-reaching consequences of anxiety and its potential to hinder personal growth.

By immersing ourselves in these foundational aspects of anxiety, we lay the groundwork for our transformative journey ahead. Remember, knowledge is power, and as we delve deeper into understanding anxiety, we become better equipped to challenge and conquer its grip.

Through personal anecdotes, expert insights, and actionable strategies, we will embark on a path of self-discovery and empowerment. Together, we will unshackle anxiety and pave the way for lasting freedom. Get ready to embark on a journey of transformation, as we discover the strategies and insights that will help you reclaim your life from anxiety's grasp. Let's begin this empowering journey together.

Note: While this book provides guidance and insights, it is important to seek professional help if you require medical or therapeutic support. The strategies discussed here are not intended to replace professional advice but rather to complement and enhance your journey towards overcoming anxiety.

In Chapter 2, we will dive deeper into the essence of anxiety and explore its multifaceted nature.

2

Defining anxiety

Anxiety is a complex and multifaceted emotion that affects countless individuals worldwide. It manifests differently for each person, encompassing a range of thoughts, feelings, and physical sensations. By delving into the definition of anxiety, we can gain a clearer understanding of its various forms and how it impacts our lives.

At its core, anxiety is a normal and natural response to perceived threats or stressful situations. It is an instinctive reaction designed to keep us safe, activating our fight-or-flight response when faced with potential danger. However, when anxiety becomes chronic or excessive, it can significantly disrupt our daily lives and hinder our well-being.

Anxiety can take on different forms, including generalized anxiety disorder (GAD), social anxiety disorder, panic disorder, specific phobias, and more. Each form carries its own unique set of symptoms and challenges. It is essential to remember that anxiety is not a character flaw or a weakness; it is a common human experience that many people face.

Some common symptoms of anxiety include persistent worry, restlessness, irritability, difficulty concentrating, muscle tension, sleep disturbances, and overwhelming fear or panic. These symptoms can vary in intensity and frequency, and they often interfere with our ability to function optimally in our personal and professional lives.

It's important to differentiate between everyday worries and clinical anxiety. While it is normal to experience occasional worry or stress, clinical anxiety persists and intensifies, significantly impacting our quality of life. Understanding the distinction can help us recognize when anxiety becomes a problem that requires our attention and intervention.

Furthermore, anxiety often coexists with other mental health conditions such as depression, obsessive-compulsive disorder (OCD), or post-traumatic stress disorder (PTSD). Recognizing these connections can provide valuable insights into the underlying mechanisms of anxiety and inform our approach to treatment and management.

By exploring the nuances and dimensions of anxiety, we can develop a deeper empathy and understanding for ourselves and others who grapple with this condition. Remember, you are not alone in your experience, and there is hope for reclaiming your life from anxiety's grip.

In the upcoming chapters, we will delve further into the causes and triggers of anxiety, as well as explore effective strategies for managing and overcoming it. By acquiring a comprehensive understanding of anxiety, we lay the foundation for personal growth, resilience, and lasting freedom.

Continue reading in Chapter 3, where we will explore the various factors that contribute to the development and maintenance of anxiety.

3

Exploring the Causes of Anxiety

Anxiety is a complex condition influenced by a multitude of factors. By exploring the causes and triggers of anxiety, we can gain valuable insights into its origins and better understand how it manifests in our lives. Let's delve into the various factors that contribute to anxiety and how they can influence our well-being.

Biological Factors

Biological factors play a significant role in anxiety. Genetics, brain chemistry, and hormonal imbalances can contribute to an individual's predisposition to anxiety. Research suggests that certain genetic variations may increase the likelihood of developing anxiety disorders. Additionally, imbalances in neurotransmitters, such as serotonin and dopamine, can impact mood regulation and anxiety levels.

Environmental Factors

Our environment plays a crucial role in shaping our experiences and influencing anxiety. Traumatic events, chronic stress, and significant life changes can trigger or exacerbate anxiety symptoms. Childhood experiences, such as abuse, neglect, or unstable family dynamics, can also contribute to the development of anxiety later in life. Furthermore, ongoing exposure to stressful environments, such as high-pressure work environments or challenging interpersonal relationships, can contribute to chronic anxiety.

Cognitive Factors

Our thoughts, beliefs, and perceptions significantly influence anxiety. Negative thinking patterns, irrational beliefs, and catastrophic thinking can fuel anxiety and perpetuate its cycle. For example, individuals with anxiety often engage in "what-if" thinking, imagining the worst-case scenarios and catastrophizing outcomes. Challenging and modifying these cognitive patterns is a crucial aspect of managing anxiety effectively.

Behavioral Factors

Our behaviors and lifestyle choices can impact anxiety levels. Avoidance behaviors, excessive reassurance-seeking, and safety-seeking behaviors can reinforce anxiety and prevent us from confronting our fears. Substance abuse, poor sleep habits, and lack of physical activity can also contribute to increased anxiety. On the other hand, adopting healthy coping mechanisms, engaging in relaxation techniques, and practicing self-care can help alleviate anxiety symptoms.

Social and Cultural Factors

Social and cultural factors can influence anxiety experiences. Cultural expectations, societal pressures, and stigma surrounding mental health can contribute to anxiety symptoms. Additionally, social support, or the lack thereof, can impact how individuals cope with anxiety. Supportive relationships and a sense of belonging can provide a buffer against anxiety, while social isolation can intensify its effects.

It's important to note that these factors interact and influence one another, contributing to the complexity of anxiety. Each individual's experience of anxiety is unique, and the underlying causes can vary. Understanding the interplay between these factors can help us develop a comprehensive approach to managing anxiety.

In the following chapters, we will explore empowering strategies and techniques to address these causes and manage anxiety effectively. By recognizing the underlying factors and triggers, we can develop personalized tools for lasting freedom from anxiety.

Continue reading in Chapter 4, where we will explore the impact of anxiety on daily life and the challenges it poses for personal growth and well-being.

4

The Impact of Anxiety on Daily Life

Anxiety has far-reaching effects that permeate various aspects of our daily lives. It can significantly impact our mental, emotional, and physical well-being, as well as hinder our personal growth and overall quality of life. In this chapter, we will explore the profound consequences of anxiety and gain insight into the challenges it poses.

Mental and Emotional Well-being

Anxiety can have a profound impact on our mental and emotional states. Persistent worry, fear, and intrusive thoughts can consume our minds, making it difficult to concentrate, think clearly, and make decisions. Anxiety may also lead to irritability, restlessness, and a heightened sense of vigilance. Over time, these symptoms can contribute to feelings of overwhelm, exhaustion, and a diminished sense of joy and fulfillment.

Relationships and Social Interactions

Anxiety can strain relationships and social interactions. It may lead to social withdrawal, avoidance of certain situations, or difficulty engaging in conversations and social activities. These behaviors can create barriers to forming and maintaining meaningful connections with others. Anxiety may also cause misunderstandings, as our heightened sensitivity can lead to overreacting or misinterpreting others' intentions.

Work and Productivity

Anxiety can significantly impact our performance and productivity at work or in our studies. Difficulty concentrating, racing thoughts, and fear of making mistakes can hinder our ability to focus and meet deadlines. Anxiety may also contribute to perfectionism, as we constantly strive to meet unrealistic standards, leading to added stress and decreased productivity.

Physical Health

Anxiety can manifest in physical symptoms and take a toll on our physical health. It may lead to muscle tension, headaches, gastrointestinal disturbances, sleep disturbances, and a compromised immune system. Chronic anxiety can also contribute to the development of other health conditions, such as cardiovascular issues or weakened immune responses.

Personal Growth and Self-esteem

Anxiety can impede personal growth and self-esteem. It may limit our willingness to take risks, explore new opportunities, or step outside of our comfort zones. Anxiety often feeds self-doubt and negative self-talk, eroding our confidence and belief in our abilities. Over time, this can hinder our personal development and prevent us from reaching our full potential.

Understanding the impact of anxiety on these various areas of our lives helps us recognize the significance of addressing and managing anxiety effectively. It emphasizes the importance of seeking support, implementing coping strategies, and developing resilience to minimize the negative consequences.

In the upcoming chapters, we will delve into empowering strategies and techniques for managing anxiety, cultivating resilience, and promoting overall well-being. By developing a comprehensive toolkit, we can navigate the challenges posed by anxiety and pave the way for personal growth, lasting freedom, and a more fulfilling life.

Continue reading in Chapter 5, where we will explore mindset shifts and perspectives that can empower us to overcome anxiety and reclaim our lives.

II

Overcoming Anxiety: Mindset Shifts

5

Shifting Perspectives on Anxiety

To overcome anxiety, it is essential to cultivate a mindset that empowers us to challenge and transcend its grip. In this chapter, we will explore transformative perspectives on anxiety that can shift our relationship with it and empower us to take control of our lives. By adopting these perspectives, we can embark on a path of self-discovery and lasting freedom.

Embracing Anxiety as a Messenger

Rather than viewing anxiety as a purely negative force, we can reframe it as a messenger, signaling unmet needs or areas of our lives that require attention. Anxiety can highlight areas where personal growth is possible and motivate us to seek solutions. By embracing anxiety as a messenger, we can engage in self-reflection and explore the underlying causes and triggers.

Recognizing Anxiety as a Normal Human Experience

Anxiety is a natural human response to stress and perceived threats. Acknowledging that anxiety is a common experience shared by many can help reduce the stigma and self-judgment surrounding it. Understanding that anxiety does not define our worth or character allows us to approach it with compassion and self-acceptance.

Reframing Anxiety as Energy for Growth

Anxiety often comes with heightened energy and a heightened sense of awareness. By reframing anxiety as energy that can be harnessed for personal growth, we can channel it into productive pursuits. This perspective allows us to view anxiety as a catalyst for change and motivates us to take positive action towards self-improvement.

Emphasizing Progress over Perfection

Anxiety often accompanies a desire for perfection and fear of making mistakes. Shifting our perspective to emphasize progress over perfection allows us to embrace a growth mindset. Recognizing that growth is a gradual process and that setbacks are natural enables us to approach challenges with resilience and learn from them, rather than being paralyzed by fear.

Viewing Anxiety as an Opportunity for Self-Compassion

Anxiety can provide an opportunity to cultivate self-compassion and kindness towards ourselves. Instead of berating ourselves for experiencing anxiety, we can offer ourselves understanding, patience, and self-care. Recognizing that everyone faces challenges and setbacks allows us to extend compassion to ourselves as we navigate the complexities of anxiety.

Seeing Anxiety as a Teacher

Anxiety can be a powerful teacher, guiding us towards self-awareness and personal transformation. By exploring the lessons that anxiety presents, we can uncover deeper insights about ourselves, our fears, and our desires. Viewing anxiety as a teacher encourages us to approach it with curiosity and openness, leading to profound self-discovery.

By adopting these perspectives on anxiety, we can reframe our relationship with it and empower ourselves to transcend its limitations. Each perspective offers a unique lens through which we can understand and navigate anxiety, fostering personal growth, resilience, and lasting freedom.

In the following chapters, we will explore practical strategies and techniques that align with these transformative perspectives. Together, we will embark on a journey of self-empowerment and discover the tools to unshackle anxiety and embrace a life of greater joy, purpose, and

Continue reading in Chapter 6, where we will delve into the practice of self-compassion as a powerful tool for managing anxiety and cultivating inner strength.

6

Embracing Self-Compassion

Self-compassion is a powerful practice that allows us to approach ourselves with kindness, understanding, and acceptance. It is an essential tool for managing anxiety and cultivating inner strength. In this chapter, we will explore the transformative practice of self-compassion and how it can support our journey towards lasting freedom from anxiety.

Understanding Self-Compassion

Self-compassion involves treating ourselves with the same kindness and care we would extend to a loved one. It encompasses three key components: self-kindness, common humanity, and mindfulness. Self-kindness entails being gentle and understanding with ourselves, especially during times of struggle. Recognizing our shared humanity reminds us that we are not alone in our experiences, and others also face challenges and setbacks. Mindfulness involves being present and non-judgmental, allowing us to observe our thoughts and emotions without self-criticism.

Letting Go of Self-Judgment

Anxiety often accompanies self-judgment and self-criticism. By cultivating self-compassion, we learn to let go of harsh self-judgment and embrace a more understanding and forgiving stance towards ourselves. Instead of berating ourselves for experiencing anxiety, we offer ourselves kindness and support. Self-compassion shifts our inner dialogue from one of self-blame to one of self-encouragement and nurturance.

Practicing Self-Kindness

Self-kindness involves actively treating ourselves with care, warmth, and understanding. It means acknowledging our struggles and difficulties without judgment. Engaging in self-soothing activities such as self-care routines, comforting rituals, or engaging in hobbies that bring us joy can foster self-kindness. Nurturing ourselves physically, emotionally, and mentally promotes a sense of safety and well-being, counteracting the grip of anxiety.

Connecting with Shared Humanity

Anxiety often leads us to feel isolated and alone in our struggles. However, embracing self-compassion reminds us that we are not alone. Recognizing our shared humanity allows us to connect with others who also experience anxiety, fostering a sense of belonging and empathy. Sharing our experiences and seeking support from others who understand can provide a powerful source of strength and reassurance.

Practicing Mindful Awareness

Mindfulness plays a crucial role in self-compassion. By practicing mindful awareness, we develop the ability to observe our thoughts and emotions without judgment. This non-judgmental stance allows us to acknowledge our anxiety without getting caught up in self-critical narratives. Mindfulness helps us cultivate self-compassion by bringing our attention to the present moment and fostering a sense of acceptance and self-acceptance.

Embracing Imperfection

Anxiety often arises from a fear of not being good enough or making mistakes. Embracing self-compassion involves recognizing that imperfection is an inherent part of being human. Instead of striving for unattainable perfection, we embrace ourselves with all our flaws and vulnerabilities. Embracing imperfection allows us to navigate anxiety with self-acceptance, celebrating our progress and growth rather than being paralyzed by self-judgment.

Practicing self-compassion is a transformative process that requires patience and gentle persistence. By embracing self-compassion, we offer ourselves the support, love, and understanding we deserve. It enables us to navigate anxiety with greater resilience, self-acceptance, and emotional well-being.

In the following chapters, we will continue our exploration of empowering strategies and techniques for managing anxiety, fostering resilience, and cultivating lasting freedom. Remember to be kind to yourself and extend the same compassion to yourself that you would offer to a cherished friend.

7

Cultivating Resilience

Resilience is a powerful trait that enables us to bounce back from adversity, navigate challenges, and thrive in the face of uncertainty. Cultivating resilience is an essential aspect of overcoming anxiety and building lasting freedom. In this chapter, we will explore strategies and practices that can help us develop resilience and strengthen our ability to navigate the ups and downs of life.

Embracing Change and Adaptability

Resilience involves embracing change as a natural part of life and developing adaptability. Change can be unsettling, but viewing it as an opportunity for growth and learning allows us to approach it with openness and flexibility. By cultivating a mindset that welcomes change, we become better equipped to navigate the uncertainties that trigger anxiety.

Building a Supportive Network

Surrounding ourselves with a supportive network of family, friends, or support groups is crucial for resilience. Cultivating connections and seeking support not only provides emotional comfort but also offers different perspectives and resources for managing anxiety. Sharing our struggles and experiences with trusted individuals can alleviate the burden of anxiety and foster resilience.

Developing Emotional Regulation Skills

Resilience involves developing effective emotional regulation skills. Learning to recognize and manage our emotions in healthy ways can help prevent anxiety from spiraling out of control. Techniques such as deep breathing exercises, mindfulness, and grounding techniques can help regulate our emotions and bring a sense of calm during times of heightened anxiety.

Cultivating Optimism and Positive Thinking

Optimism and positive thinking contribute to resilience by fostering a mindset that focuses on possibilities and solutions. Embracing a positive outlook does not mean ignoring challenges or denying the existence of anxiety, but rather acknowledging difficulties while maintaining faith in our ability to overcome them. Positive affirmations, gratitude practices, and reframing negative thoughts can help shift our perspective towards optimism.

Practicing Self-Care and Stress Management

Prioritizing self-care is vital for building resilience. Engaging in activities that promote relaxation, joy, and well-being helps restore our physical and mental energy. Adequate sleep, regular exercise, healthy nutrition, and engaging in hobbies or creative outlets can reduce stress and enhance our ability to cope with anxiety. Taking time for self-reflection and setting boundaries also contribute to self-care and resilience.

Cultivating a Growth Mindset

Resilience is closely tied to adopting a growth mindset—a belief that our abilities and intelligence can be developed through effort and learning. Embracing challenges, reframing setbacks as opportunities for growth, and seeking continuous personal development foster resilience. By cultivating a growth mindset, we can approach anxiety as an opportunity for self-improvement and navigate it with determination and resilience.

Practicing Self-Compassion

Self-compassion is an essential component of resilience. Showing ourselves kindness, understanding, and acceptance during difficult times allows us to bounce back from setbacks with greater strength. Embracing self-compassion means acknowledging that experiencing anxiety is a normal human experience and treating ourselves with the same compassion we would extend to a friend facing similar challenges.

Cultivating resilience is an ongoing journey that requires practice and dedication. By incorporating these strategies into our lives, we can develop resilience and fortify ourselves against the impact of anxiety. Remember that resilience is not about avoiding challenges but rather about building the inner strength and tools to navigate them with grace and determination.

In the following chapters, we will continue to explore empowering strategies and techniques that foster resilience and support our journey toward lasting freedom from anxiety.

8

Managing Negative Thoughts and Beliefs

Negative thoughts and beliefs can contribute to anxiety and hinder our well-being. In this chapter, we will explore effective strategies for managing and challenging negative thinking patterns. By cultivating awareness and developing healthier thought patterns, we can free ourselves from the grip of anxiety and cultivate a more positive and empowered

Recognizing Negative Thought Patterns

The first step in managing negative thoughts is to become aware of them. Pay attention to the stream of thoughts that arise in your mind, particularly those that contribute to anxiety. Common negative thought patterns include catastrophic thinking (assuming the worst-case scenario), black-and-white thinking (seeing things in extremes), and overgeneralization (drawing sweeping conclusions based on limited evidence). By recognizing these patterns, you can interrupt their influence on your emotions and behavior.

Questioning the Validity of Negative Thoughts

Once you've identified negative thoughts, it's important to question their validity. Ask yourself if there is concrete evidence supporting the negative thought or if it's based on assumptions or irrational fears. Challenge the accuracy of the negative thought and explore alternative perspectives or explanations. Often, negative thoughts are distorted and do not reflect reality. By questioning their validity, you can weaken their power over you.

Reframing Negative Thoughts

Reframing involves shifting the perspective of a negative thought to a more balanced and realistic viewpoint. Look for evidence that contradicts the negative thought and consider alternative explanations or interpretations. For example, if your negative thought is "I'm always going to fail," reframe it to "I've had successes in the past, and failure is a natural part of growth and learning." Reframing helps to broaden your perspective and create more positive and constructive thought patterns.

Practicing Cognitive Restructuring

Cognitive restructuring is a technique that involves actively replacing negative thoughts with more positive and rational ones. When a negative thought arises, challenge it and replace it with a more balanced and empowering thought. For instance, if your negative thought is "I can't handle this," restructure it to "I may feel anxious, but I have successfully coped with challenging situations before, and I can handle this too." Practice this technique consistently to rewire your thought patterns over time.

Utilizing Thought-Stopping Techniques

Thought-stopping techniques help interrupt and redirect the flow of negative thoughts. When you notice a negative thought arising, mentally say "Stop!" or use a physical gesture like snapping a rubber band on your wrist. Then, consciously replace the negative thought with a more positive or neutral thought. This technique breaks the automatic cycle of negative thinking and creates space for more constructive thoughts to emerge.

Cultivating Self-Compassionate Inner Dialogue

Replace self-critical inner dialogue with self-compassionate and supportive thoughts. Treat yourself with kindness and understanding, just as you would offer support to a friend facing similar challenges. Remind yourself that anxiety is a normal experience and that you are doing your best. Engage in positive self-talk, affirmations, and reminders of your strengths and past successes.

Engaging in Mindfulness Practices

Mindfulness can help you observe negative thoughts without getting caught up in them. Practice being present in the moment and observe your thoughts without judgment. When negative thoughts arise, acknowledge them and let them pass without getting entangled in their content. Mindfulness cultivates a sense of detachment from negative thoughts, allowing you to create space for more positive and empowering thoughts to arise.

Managing negative thoughts and beliefs requires consistent effort and practice. By implementing these strategies, you can gain greater control over your thought patterns, reduce anxiety, and cultivate a more positive and empowered mindset. Remember that challenging negative thoughts takes time and patience, so be gentle with yourself as you work towards rewiring your thinking patterns.

In the following chapters, we will continue our exploration of empowering strategies and techniques for managing anxiety and achieving lasting freedom.

III

Empowering strategies for managing anxiety

9

Breathing Techniques and Mindfulness Practices

Breathing techniques and mindfulness practices are powerful tools for managing anxiety and cultivating a sense of calm and centeredness. In this chapter, we will explore various techniques that can help regulate your breathing and bring mindfulness into your daily life. By incorporating these practices into your routine, you can find relief from anxiety and develop greater resilience.

Deep Abdominal Breathing

Deep abdominal breathing, also known as diaphragmatic breathing, is a simple yet effective technique for calming the body and mind. Find a comfortable seated or lying position and place one hand on your abdomen. Breathe in deeply through your nose, allowing your abdomen to rise as you fill your lungs with air. Exhale slowly through your mouth, feeling your abdomen gently deflate. Focus on the sensation of your breath, and repeat this cycle several times, allowing each breath to bring a sense of relaxation and grounding.

Box Breathing

Box breathing is a technique that promotes relaxation and balances the autonomic nervous system. Visualize a box shape in your mind. Inhale deeply through your nose for a count of four, envisioning the upward line of the box. Hold your breath for a count of four, visualizing the line across the top of the box. Exhale slowly through your mouth for a count of four, envisioning the downward line of the box. Finally, hold your breath for a count of four, completing the box shape. Repeat this cycle several times, synchronizing your breath with the visualized box, and notice the calming effect it brings.

Mindful Breathing

Mindful breathing involves bringing full attention to your breath as it naturally flows in and out. Find a comfortable position and focus your attention on the sensation of your breath entering and leaving your body. Observe the rising and falling of your abdomen or the sensation of air passing through your nostrils. When your mind wanders, gently bring your attention back to your breath, without judgment. Practice this mindful breathing for a few minutes each day, gradually increasing the duration as you become more comfortable with the practice.

Body Scan Meditation

Body scan meditation is a practice that promotes body awareness and relaxation. Find a quiet and comfortable space to lie down. Starting from your toes, bring your attention to each part of your body, moving upward gradually. Notice any sensations, tension, or areas of relaxation as you scan through your body. Breathe into any areas of tension, allowing them to release with each exhale. This practice helps you develop a deeper connection with your body and promotes relaxation and grounding.

Mindfulness in Daily Activities

Incorporating mindfulness into your daily activities can be a powerful way to cultivate present-moment awareness and reduce anxiety. Choose a routine activity, such as washing dishes, taking a shower, or walking, and bring your full attention to the sensory experience of that activity. Notice the temperature of the water, the scent of the soap, the sensation of your feet touching the ground. Whenever your mind drifts to anxious thoughts, gently guide it back to the present moment and the sensory experience at hand.

Loving-Kindness Meditation

Loving-kindness meditation is a practice that cultivates compassion and kindness towards yourself and others. Find a quiet and comfortable space to sit. Begin by directing loving and kind phrases towards yourself, such as "May I be safe, may I be happy, may I be healthy, may I live with ease." Then extend these phrases to loved ones, acquaintances, neutral people, and even difficult individuals. This practice fosters a sense of connection, empathy, and kindness, helping to counteract anxiety and promote a more positive mindset.

By incorporating breathing techniques and mindfulness practices into your life, you can create moments of calm and develop a greater capacity to manage anxiety. These practices offer a way to cultivate present-moment awareness, regulate your breathing, and nurture a more compassionate relationship with yourself and the world around you.

In the following chapters, we will continue exploring empowering strategies and techniques for managing anxiety, cultivating well-being, and achieving lasting freedom.

10

The Power of Visualization and Imagery

Visualization and imagery techniques tap into the power of the mind to create positive mental images and evoke soothing sensory experiences. In this chapter, we will explore how visualization and imagery can be harnessed to manage anxiety and promote a sense of calm and well-being. By incorporating these techniques into your practice, you can harness the power of your imagination to support your journey towards lasting freedom.

Guided Visualization

Guided visualization involves creating vivid mental images that evoke a sense of calm and relaxation. Find a quiet and comfortable space to sit or lie down. Close your eyes and imagine yourself in a peaceful and serene setting, such as a beach, a lush forest, or a tranquil garden. Engage all your senses in this visualization—feel the warmth of the sun, hear the soothing sounds of nature, and smell the fragrant flowers. Allow yourself to fully immerse in this mental imagery, experiencing a profound sense of tranquility and peace.

Positive Future Visualization

Positive future visualization focuses on envisioning positive outcomes and experiences. Close your eyes and visualize yourself engaging in activities that bring you joy, accomplishing your goals, and overcoming challenges with confidence. Create a detailed mental picture of your desired future, including the emotions and sensations associated with it. As you immerse yourself in this visualization, allow the positive feelings to permeate your being, cultivating a sense of optimism and empowerment.

Safe Place Imagery

Safe place imagery involves creating a mental sanctuary where you feel safe, calm, and protected. Visualize a place that brings you a deep sense of comfort and security—it can be a real or imagined location. It could be a cozy room, a beautiful garden, or a tranquil lakeside. Engage your senses and immerse yourself in this mental image, focusing on the soothing qualities of the environment. Whenever you feel anxious or overwhelmed, imagine yourself in this safe place, drawing upon its calming energy to alleviate anxiety.

Breath Visualization

Breath visualization combines deep breathing techniques with imagery to enhance relaxation and focus. As you engage in deep abdominal breathing, visualize your breath as a soothing color or light. Imagine that with each inhalation, you are drawing in this calming color or light, and with each exhalation, you are releasing any tension or anxiety, allowing it to dissipate. Sync your breath with the visualization, using it as an anchor to bring your attention to the present moment and promote a sense of calm.

Mental Rehearsal

Mental rehearsal involves visualizing yourself successfully navigating challenging situations or overcoming anxiety-inducing scenarios. Before confronting a feared situation or engaging in a stressful task, take a few moments to mentally rehearse yourself handling it with confidence and ease. Visualize the desired outcome, envisioning yourself managing the situation effectively and feeling calm and in control. This technique can help reduce anxiety and enhance your belief in your ability to handle challenging circumstances.

Affirmation Visualization

Affirmation visualization combines positive affirmations with imagery to reinforce empowering beliefs and attitudes. Create a positive affirmation that resonates with you, such as "I am calm and capable in the face of challenges." Close your eyes and repeat this affirmation to yourself while visualizing it coming to life. Imagine the affirmation as a vibrant, glowing script or picture that surrounds you, filling you with its positive energy and strengthening your belief in your resilience and ability to overcome anxiety.

Visualization and imagery techniques harness the power of your imagination to create a sense of calm, positivity, and empowerment. Incorporating these techniques into your practice can help reduce anxiety, promote relaxation, and enhance your overall well-being.

In the following chapters, we will continue exploring empowering strategies and techniques for managing anxiety, cultivating resilience, and achieving lasting freedom.

11

Exercise and Physical Well-being

Physical activity and exercise are powerful tools for managing anxiety and promoting overall well-being. In this chapter, we will explore the benefits of exercise and strategies for incorporating it into your routine. By prioritizing exercise and nurturing your physical well-being, you can reduce anxiety, boost your mood, and enhance your resilience.

Benefits of Exercise for Anxiety

Engaging in regular exercise has numerous benefits for anxiety management. Physical activity releases endorphins, which are natural mood-boosting chemicals in the brain, promoting a sense of well-being and reducing anxiety. Exercise also helps to reduce muscle tension and promote relaxation, alleviating physical symptoms associated with anxiety. Additionally, regular exercise improves sleep quality, increases energy levels, and enhances overall resilience to stress.

Finding an Exercise Routine

Choose an exercise routine that suits your preferences and fits into your lifestyle. It could be aerobic activities such as walking, running, swimming, or cycling that elevate your heart rate and increase oxygen flow. Alternatively, you may enjoy activities like yoga, Pilates, or tai chi, which combine physical movement with mindfulness and relaxation techniques. Experiment with different forms of exercise to find what resonates with you and brings you joy.

Creating Consistency

Consistency is key to reaping the benefits of exercise for anxiety management. Set realistic goals and create a schedule that allows for regular physical activity. Start with manageable durations and gradually increase intensity or duration as your fitness level improves. Aim for at least 150 minutes of moderate-intensity aerobic activity per week, or 75 minutes of vigorous-intensity activity. Remember, even short bursts of exercise can be beneficial, so find opportunities to be active throughout your day.

Mindful Movement

Practice mindful movement during exercise by bringing your full attention to the sensations in your body as you move. Notice your breath, the rhythm of your steps or movements, and the feeling of your muscles working. Engage in the present moment, allowing exercise to become a form of moving meditation. Mindful movement enhances the mind–body connection, promoting a sense of calm and grounding.

Outdoor Activities and Nature

Incorporating outdoor activities and spending time in nature can amplify the benefits of exercise for anxiety management. Nature has a soothing effect on the mind and helps reduce stress. Whether it's going for a hike, practicing yoga in the park, or simply taking a walk in a natural setting, immersing yourself in nature adds an extra dimension of relaxation and connection with the world around you.

Social Engagement through Exercise

Engaging in exercise with others can enhance the positive effects on anxiety management. Joining group fitness classes, team sports, or exercising with a friend or loved one provides an opportunity for social connection and support. Sharing the exercise experience with others can boost motivation, provide accountability, and foster a sense of camaraderie, reducing feelings of isolation and anxiety.

Listen to Your Body

Pay attention to your body's signals during exercise. Respect your limits and modify activities as needed. Push yourself within a comfortable range, but avoid overexertion, which can increase stress and anxiety. Be mindful of any physical conditions or injuries, and seek guidance from healthcare professionals or fitness experts if necessary.

By incorporating exercise and physical well-being into your life, you can harness the natural benefits of movement to manage anxiety and promote a greater sense of well-being. Prioritize your physical health, engage in activities that bring you joy, and listen to your body's needs.

In the following chapters, we will continue exploring empowering strategies and techniques for managing anxiety, fostering resilience, and achieving lasting freedom.

12

Harnessing the Benefits of Journaling and Self-Reflection

Journaling and self-reflection are powerful practices that can support anxiety management, self-awareness, and personal growth. In this chapter, we will explore the benefits of journaling and techniques for incorporating self-reflection into your daily life. By engaging in these practices, you can gain clarity, process emotions, and cultivate a deeper understanding of yourself, leading to greater resilience and lasting freedom.

The Power of Journaling

Journaling provides a safe and private space for self-expression and exploration. It allows you to externalize your thoughts and emotions, gaining perspective and insight into your experiences. The act of putting pen to paper can be cathartic and therapeutic, helping to release pent-up emotions and reduce anxiety. Journaling also serves as a valuable record of your journey, allowing you to track progress and identify patterns or triggers related to your anxiety.

Freewriting

Freewriting is a technique that involves writing without constraints or self-censorship. Set a timer for a designated period, such as 10 to 15 minutes, and let your thoughts flow onto the pages without judgment or the need to edit. Write whatever comes to mind, allowing your thoughts and feelings to spill onto the paper. This practice promotes self-expression and can help uncover underlying emotions and insights.

Gratitude Journaling

Gratitude journaling involves writing down things you are grateful for each day. Set aside a few minutes each day to reflect on the positive aspects of your life and write them down in your journal. This practice shifts your focus towards gratitude and appreciation, fostering a positive mindset and reducing anxiety. Regularly acknowledging the good in your life can counterbalance negative thoughts and emotions.

Emotion Journaling

Emotion journaling focuses on exploring and processing your emotions. When you experience anxiety or intense emotions, take a moment to sit with those feelings and then write about them in your journal. Describe the emotions, their intensity, and any accompanying physical sensations. Reflect on the possible triggers or underlying causes of these emotions. This practice allows you to gain clarity, release emotions, and develop a deeper understanding of yourself.

Self-Reflection Prompts

Utilize self-reflection prompts to guide your journaling practice. These prompts can encourage self-exploration and insight. Some examples include:

- "What are my biggest sources of anxiety, and how do they impact my daily life?"
- "What strategies have worked for me in managing anxiety in the past?"
- "What self-care practices or activities bring me a sense of calm and joy?"
- "What limiting beliefs or negative thought patterns contribute to my anxiety, and how can I challenge them?"
- "What are my strengths and positive qualities that can support me in overcoming anxiety?"

Writing Affirmations

Affirmations are positive statements that can help shift your mindset and counteract negative self-talk. Write affirmations that resonate with you and address your specific anxiety challenges. For example, "I am capable of managing my anxiety with grace and resilience." Repeat these affirmations daily, either in your journal or aloud, to reinforce positive beliefs and empower yourself.

Reflection on Growth and Progress

Regularly reflect on your growth and progress in managing anxiety. Look back at previous journal entries and notice the changes, insights, and milestones you have achieved. Celebrate your accomplishments and acknowledge your resilience. Reflection on growth reinforces your ability to overcome challenges and builds confidence in your journey towards lasting freedom.

Journaling and self-reflection offer valuable avenues for self-discovery, emotional processing, and personal growth. They provide a means of understanding your anxiety, uncovering patterns, and developing strategies for managing it effectively.

In the following chapters, we will continue exploring empowering strategies and techniques for managing anxiety, cultivating resilience, and achieving lasting freedom.

IV

Building a Supportive Lifestyle

13

Nurturing Relationships and Connection

Strong and supportive relationships play a vital role in managing anxiety and promoting overall well-being. In this chapter, we will explore the importance of nurturing relationships and techniques for fostering meaningful connections. By prioritizing healthy relationships in your life, you can cultivate a support system that contributes to your journey towards lasting freedom.

Recognizing the Importance of Relationships

Relationships provide emotional support, companionship, and a sense of belonging, all of which are crucial for managing anxiety. Acknowledge the significance of relationships in your life and the impact they have on your mental and emotional well-being. Cultivating strong connections can provide a buffer against anxiety, offering comfort, understanding, and encouragement.

Communicating Openly and Honestly

Effective communication is the foundation of healthy relationships. Practice open and honest communication with your loved ones, expressing your needs, concerns, and feelings. Be attentive and compassionate listeners when others share their experiences and emotions. Open communication fosters understanding, strengthens bonds, and helps build a network of support.

Prioritizing Quality Time

Allocate dedicated time to spend with your loved ones and engage in meaningful activities together. This can involve shared hobbies, going for walks, having meaningful conversations, or simply enjoying each other's company. Quality time nurtures connections and creates opportunities for bonding and support.

Seeking Emotional Support

Don't hesitate to reach out for emotional support when you're feeling anxious. Share your experiences and feelings with trusted friends, family members, or support groups. Opening up allows others to provide comfort, perspective, and reassurance. Remember that seeking support is not a sign of weakness but a courageous act that strengthens relationships.

Setting Boundaries

Setting boundaries is essential for maintaining healthy relationships and managing anxiety. Clearly communicate your limits and needs to ensure that your relationships are mutually respectful and supportive. Recognize when you need personal space or time to recharge, and communicate this openly. Setting boundaries ensures that your relationships are balanced and conducive to your well-being.

Cultivating Empathy and Compassion

Practice empathy and compassion towards yourself and others. Seek to understand the experiences and emotions of those around you, and offer support and kindness. Foster an environment of empathy and compassion within your relationships, creating a safe space for vulnerability and growth.

Engaging in Acts of Kindness

Engage in acts of kindness towards your loved ones and the broader community. Small gestures of kindness, such as a thoughtful note, a helping hand, or a kind word, can have a significant positive impact on your relationships. By fostering a culture of kindness, you contribute to a supportive and uplifting social network.

Embracing Diversity and Connection

Embrace diversity and seek connections with individuals from different backgrounds, experiences, and perspectives. Engaging with diverse communities broadens your understanding, challenges preconceived notions, and fosters personal growth. Cultivate an inclusive mindset and create opportunities for connection with people who expand your horizons.

Balancing Online and Offline Interactions

In today's digital age, it's important to strike a balance between online and offline interactions. While online connections can be valuable, prioritize face-to-face interactions whenever possible. Engage in meaningful conversations and nurture deep connections that go beyond superficial interactions.

Nurturing relationships and connections is a lifelong journey that requires time, effort, and genuine care. By investing in healthy and supportive relationships, you create a network of individuals who can provide understanding, encouragement, and strength as you navigate anxiety and pursue lasting freedom.

In the following chapters, we will continue exploring empowering strategies and techniques for managing anxiety, cultivating resilience, and achieving lasting freedom.

14

Setting Boundaries and Prioritizing Self-Care

Setting boundaries and prioritizing self-care are vital components of managing anxiety and fostering a healthy and balanced lifestyle. In this chapter, we will explore the importance of establishing boundaries and techniques for prioritizing self-care. By honoring your needs and creating healthy boundaries, you can cultivate well-being, reduce anxiety, and achieve lasting freedom.

Understanding Boundaries

Boundaries are the limits we set for ourselves in various areas of our lives to protect our well-being and honor our needs. They define what is acceptable and what is not in terms of our time, energy, and emotional investment. Recognize that setting boundaries is an act of self-respect and self-care.

Identifying Your Needs

Take time to identify your personal needs and values. Reflect on what is important to you and what supports your well-being. This may include alone time, rest, meaningful connections, pursuing your passions, or maintaining a healthy work-life balance. Understanding your needs allows you to set boundaries that align with your values and priorities.

Establishing Clear Communication

Communicate your boundaries effectively and assertively with others. Clearly express your needs, limits, and expectations in a respectful manner. Use "I" statements to express how certain behaviors or situations impact you. Practice open and honest communication, and remember that you have the right to establish boundaries that promote your well-being.

Learning to Say No

Saying no is a powerful act of self-care. It allows you to prioritize your needs and protect your time and energy. Practice saying no without guilt or apology when requests or obligations do not align with your boundaries or priorities. Remember that saying no to others means saying yes to yourself and your well-being.

Managing Time and Energy

Effectively manage your time and energy by establishing boundaries around how you allocate them. Prioritize activities and relationships that bring you joy, fulfillment, and support your well-being. Set realistic expectations for yourself and avoid overcommitting or overextending yourself. Consider using time management techniques such as prioritizing tasks, delegating when possible, and scheduling regular breaks for self-care.

Creating Digital Boundaries

In today's digital age, it's essential to establish boundaries around technology use. Set limits on screen time, establish technology-free zones or times, and be intentional about engaging in activities that nourish your well-being offline. Practice being fully present in the moment and disconnecting from digital distractions when needed.

Self-Care as a Priority

Prioritize self-care as an essential aspect of your daily life. Incorporate self-care activities into your routine and allocate dedicated time for self-care practices that nurture your physical, mental, and emotional well-being. Treat self-care as a non-negotiable commitment to yourself, just as you would prioritize other important responsibilities.

Self-Compassion and Self-Kindness

Practice self-compassion and self-kindness as you set boundaries and prioritize self-care. Be gentle with yourself and acknowledge that it's okay to put yourself first. Release any guilt or judgment surrounding your self-care practices, understanding that taking care of yourself enables you to show up fully in other areas of your life.

Regular Evaluation and Adjustments

Regularly evaluate your boundaries and self-care practices to ensure they align with your evolving needs and circumstances. Check-in with yourself and make adjustments as necessary. Be flexible and open to refining your boundaries and self-care routines based on your growth and changing priorities.

Setting boundaries and prioritizing self-care empower you to create a life that supports your well-being and manages anxiety effectively. By establishing healthy limits and honoring your needs, you cultivate a nurturing and balanced lifestyle.

In the following chapters, we will continue exploring empowering strategies and techniques for managing anxiety, fostering resilience, and achieving lasting freedom.

15

Creating a Calming Environment

Your physical environment has a significant impact on your overall well-being and can greatly influence your anxiety levels. In this chapter, we will explore techniques for creating a calming environment that supports your journey towards lasting freedom from anxiety. By intentionally designing your surroundings, you can promote relaxation, reduce stress, and cultivate a sense of tranquility.

Declutter and Organize

Begin by decluttering and organizing your physical space. Clutter can contribute to feelings of overwhelm and anxiety. Take the time to sort through your belongings, identifying items you no longer need or that no longer serve you. Create a system for organizing your space that suits your preferences and promotes a sense of order and simplicity.

Calming Colors and Lighting

Choose colors that promote a sense of calm and relaxation in your environment. Soft, neutral tones like pastels or earthy shades can create a soothing atmosphere. Consider incorporating natural light whenever possible or use warm, gentle lighting to create a cozy and inviting ambiance.

Natural Elements

Bring elements of nature into your environment to evoke a sense of tranquility. Incorporate plants, flowers, or natural materials like wood and stone. Spending time in the presence of nature, even indoors, can have a calming effect on your mind and body.

Sensory Soothing

Engage your senses in creating a calming environment. Incorporate soothing scents, such as aromatherapy diffusers or candles with relaxing essential oils like lavender or chamomile. Play calming background music or nature sounds to create a serene auditory atmosphere. Consider soft textures, like plush blankets or comfortable pillows, to enhance the tactile sense of coziness.

Personal Sanctuary

Designate a specific area in your home as a personal sanctuary—a space solely dedicated to relaxation and tranquility. It could be a cozy corner with a comfortable chair, a meditation cushion, or a soft rug. Personalize this space with items that bring you joy and peace, such as favorite books, inspirational quotes, or sentimental objects.

Minimize Digital Distractions

Create boundaries around technology use to reduce digital distractions and promote a calming environment. Set specific times or areas where electronic devices are not allowed. Designate technology-free zones, such as your bedroom or a particular room, to create sacred spaces free from constant notifications and distractions.

Noise Management

Manage noise levels to create a serene environment. Use noise-cancelling headphones or soft earplugs to block out unwanted sounds when necessary. Incorporate white noise machines, calming music, or nature sounds to create a soothing auditory atmosphere.

Visual Serenity

Curate your surroundings to promote visual serenity. Keep your space clean, organized, and free from visual clutter. Display artwork, photographs, or images that evoke a sense of calm and joy. Consider incorporating elements of symmetry and balance in your decor to create visual harmony.

Personalize Your Space

Infuse your environment with personal touches that bring you comfort and joy. Display cherished items, mementos, or photographs that hold positive memories. Surround yourself with objects and artwork that resonate with your values and aspirations.

Creating a calming environment is a deliberate and ongoing process. Regularly assess your surroundings and make adjustments as needed to ensure they align with your desire for tranquility and relaxation. By intentionally designing your physical environment, you can create a supportive space that nurtures your well-being and helps manage anxiety effectively.

In the following chapters, we will continue exploring empowering strategies and techniques for managing anxiety, fostering resilience, and achieving lasting freedom.

16

Managing Stress and Building Emotional Resilience

Stress is a natural part of life, but how we manage it greatly impacts our well-being and ability to navigate anxiety. In this chapter, we will explore techniques for effectively managing stress and building emotional resilience. By developing healthy coping mechanisms and cultivating resilience, you can navigate stressful situations with greater ease and achieve lasting freedom from anxiety.

Understanding Stress

Begin by understanding the nature of stress and its effects on your mind and body. Recognize the signs of stress, such as increased heart rate, muscle tension, irritability, or difficulty concentrating. Become aware of your personal stress triggers and patterns, as this self-awareness is essential in managing stress effectively.

Stress Reduction Techniques

Engage in stress reduction techniques to actively counter the effects of stress. Explore different strategies, such as deep breathing exercises, progressive muscle relaxation, or guided imagery, to elicit the relaxation response in your body. Find what works best for you and incorporate these techniques into your daily routine to proactively manage stress.

Time Management and Prioritization

Effective time management and prioritization play a crucial role in stress management. Organize your tasks, responsibilities, and commitments in a way that reduces overwhelm and allows for a sense of control. Prioritize essential activities and let go of non-essential tasks that may add unnecessary stress. Break larger tasks into smaller, manageable steps to make them more achievable and less daunting.

Healthy Lifestyle Habits

Cultivate healthy lifestyle habits that support stress management and emotional resilience. Focus on getting sufficient sleep, maintaining a balanced diet, and engaging in regular physical activity. These foundational pillars contribute to overall well-being, boost mood, and enhance your ability to cope with stress.

Mindfulness and Present-Moment Awareness

Practice mindfulness and present-moment awareness as tools for stress management. Cultivate the ability to observe your thoughts, emotions, and bodily sensations without judgment. Stay present in the moment, rather than dwelling on the past or worrying about the future. Mindfulness allows you to respond to stressors more skillfully and with greater clarity.

Positive Coping Mechanisms

Develop positive coping mechanisms for managing stress. Engage in activities that bring you joy, such as hobbies, creative outlets, or spending time with loved ones. Seek social support when needed, as sharing your concerns and feelings with trusted individuals can alleviate stress. Avoid unhealthy coping mechanisms, such as excessive alcohol or substance use, as they can exacerbate anxiety and stress in the long run.

Building Emotional Resilience

Emotional resilience is the ability to adapt and bounce back from challenging situations. Cultivate emotional resilience by reframing negative experiences, practicing self-compassion, and nurturing a positive mindset. Focus on your strengths and past successes, using them as reminders of your ability to overcome adversity. Embrace challenges as opportunities for growth and learning.

Seeking Support

Reach out for support when you're feeling overwhelmed by stress. Lean on your support network, whether it's friends, family, or professionals. Sharing your thoughts and emotions with others can provide comfort, perspective, and new insights. Consider joining support groups or seeking therapy to enhance your coping skills and build emotional resilience.

Self-Reflection and Growth

Regularly engage in self-reflection and growth as part of your stress management practice. Reflect on how you have navigated stressful situations in the past and identify areas for improvement. Learn from your experiences and actively work on developing new skills and strategies to better manage stress. Embrace a growth mindset, viewing challenges as opportunities for personal development.

Managing stress and building emotional resilience are ongoing processes that require attention and practice. By incorporating stress reduction techniques, prioritizing self-care, and fostering emotional resilience, you can navigate stressors with greater ease and create a solid foundation for managing anxiety effectively.

In the following chapters, we will continue exploring empowering strategies and techniques for managing anxiety, fostering resilience, and achieving lasting freedom.

V

Thriving Beyond Anxiety

17

Discovering Your Passions and Purpose

Thriving beyond anxiety involves connecting with your passions and living a life aligned with your purpose. In this chapter, we will explore the significance of discovering your passions and purpose and techniques for uncovering them. By embracing what truly lights you up and living with intention, you can cultivate a fulfilling and purpose-driven life beyond anxiety.

The Power of Passions and Purpose

Passions are the activities, interests, or hobbies that ignite your enthusiasm and bring you joy. Purpose is the sense of meaning and fulfillment derived from aligning your actions with your values and contributing to something greater than yourself. Discovering and embracing your passions and purpose can bring a deep sense of fulfillment and help manage anxiety by providing a sense of direction and motivation.

Reflecting on Your Interests

Begin by reflecting on your interests and what activities bring you joy and excitement. Ask yourself what makes you come alive, what you could do for hours without feeling drained, and what brings you a deep sense of satisfaction. Identify the hobbies, subjects, or areas of knowledge that captivate your attention and pique your curiosity.

Exploring New Activities

Step out of your comfort zone and explore new activities or areas of interest. Engage in experiences that you've been curious about but haven't pursued yet. This could involve taking classes, attending workshops or seminars, or simply experimenting with different hobbies. Embrace the mindset of a lifelong learner, allowing yourself to discover new passions along the way.

Pay Attention to Flow States:

Notice the activities in which you experience a state of flow—a state of complete immersion, focus, and enjoyment. Flow states occur when your skills and challenges are well-matched, allowing you to lose track of time and be fully present in the activity. Pay attention to these moments, as they can indicate areas of passion and interest.

Identify Your Values

Reflect on your core values and what is truly important to you. Your passions and purpose often align with your values. Consider what you deeply care about, whether it's creativity, compassion, growth, justice, or any other values that resonate with you. Aligning your actions with your values can bring a sense of purpose and fulfillment.

Seeking Inspiration

Seek inspiration from others who are living passionate and purpose-driven lives. Read books, watch documentaries, or listen to podcasts that explore the journeys and insights of individuals who have found their passions and purpose. Engage in conversations with mentors or role models who can provide guidance and inspire you to uncover your own passions and purpose.

Embracing Curiosity

Cultivate a mindset of curiosity and openness to the world around you. Approach each day with a sense of wonder and exploration. Ask questions, seek new experiences, and allow yourself to be curious about various subjects and activities. Curiosity fuels the journey of discovering passions and purpose.

Experiment and Refine

that the process of discovering passions and purpose is a journey of self-discovery and experimentation. Allow yourself to try different activities, explore diverse interests, and be open to evolving along the way. Embrace the process of refinement as you gain clarity on what truly resonates with you.

Taking Aligned Action

Once you have discovered your passions and aligned them with your purpose, take intentional action to incorporate them into your life. Set goals, make plans, and commit to pursuing your passions in a way that aligns with your values and purpose. Embrace challenges as opportunities for growth and allow your passions and purpose to guide your decisions and actions.

Discovering your passions and purpose is a lifelong journey. Embrace the process of exploration and self-discovery, allowing yourself to evolve and adapt along the way. By connecting with your passions and living a life aligned with your purpose, you can cultivate a sense of fulfillment, joy, and lasting freedom from anxiety.

In the following chapters, we will continue exploring empowering strategies and techniques for managing anxiety, fostering resilience, and achieving lasting freedom.

18

Cultivating Gratitude and Mindful Living

Practicing gratitude and mindful living are transformative approaches that can enhance your well-being and help you thrive beyond anxiety. In this chapter, we will explore the power of gratitude and techniques for cultivating mindfulness in your daily life. By adopting these practices, you can cultivate a greater sense of contentment, reduce anxiety, and embrace the present moment with clarity and appreciation.

The Power of Gratitude

Gratitude is the practice of acknowledging and appreciating the blessings and positive aspects of your life. It shifts your focus from what's lacking to what you already have, fostering a sense of abundance and well-being. Embracing gratitude can lead to increased happiness, resilience, and a reduction in anxiety.

Gratitude Journaling

Start a gratitude journal and make it a habit to write down things you are grateful for each day. Reflect on the simple joys, meaningful connections, and positive experiences in your life. Engaging in gratitude journaling encourages a mindset of appreciation and trains your mind to notice and savor the positive aspects of each day.

Gratitude Rituals

Incorporate gratitude rituals into your daily routine. These can include expressing gratitude aloud before meals, writing thank-you notes to express appreciation, or sharing moments of gratitude with loved ones. Embrace these rituals as opportunities to consciously cultivate gratitude and deepen your connection with others.

Shifting Perspective

Practice reframing challenges and difficulties as opportunities for growth and learning. Instead of dwelling on negative aspects, seek the lessons or silver linings within challenging situations. Shifting your perspective allows you to cultivate gratitude even during times of adversity.

Mindful Living

Mindfulness is the practice of being fully present in the moment, without judgment. It involves directing your attention to the sensations, thoughts, and emotions that arise in the present moment. By cultivating mindfulness, you can reduce anxiety, enhance self-awareness, and appreciate the richness of each experience.

Mindful Breathing

Engage in mindful breathing exercises to anchor yourself in the present moment. Focus on your breath, observing the inhale and exhale without judgment. As thoughts arise, gently bring your attention back to the breath. This practice cultivates a calm and centered state of mind, reducing anxiety and promoting clarity.

Mindful Daily Activities

Infuse mindfulness into your daily activities. Whether it's eating, walking, or washing dishes, bring your full attention to the present moment. Engage your senses and notice the sensations, smells, tastes, and sounds associated with each activity. By being fully present, you can cultivate a sense of gratitude for the simple pleasures of life.

Mindful Communication

Practice mindful communication by listening attentively and responding with presence. Be fully present and attentive when engaging in conversations with others. Notice and acknowledge their words, feelings, and non-verbal cues. Mindful communication fosters connection, understanding, and empathy.

Gratitude and Mindfulness Reminders

Place visual reminders of gratitude and mindfulness in your environment. Display meaningful quotes, images, or objects that serve as cues to pause, breathe, and cultivate gratitude and mindfulness throughout the day. These reminders can support your intention to live with gratitude and mindfulness.

Cultivating gratitude and mindful living requires practice and commitment. Embrace these practices as a way of life, allowing them to permeate your thoughts, actions, and interactions with others. By nurturing gratitude and mindfulness, you can experience a profound shift in perspective, find peace in the present moment, and thrive beyond anxiety.

In the following chapters, we will continue exploring empowering strategies and techniques for managing anxiety, fostering resilience, and achieving lasting freedom.

19

Embracing Change and Taking Risks

In this chapter, we delve into the transformative power of embracing change and taking risks as we continue our journey towards lasting freedom. Change is an inevitable part of life, and while it may often be accompanied by uncertainty and anxiety, it also holds tremendous opportunities for growth, self-discovery, and personal fulfillment. By developing a mindset that embraces change and by stepping outside our comfort zones, we open ourselves up to new possibilities and pave the way for lasting transformation.

The Nature of Change

Change is a constant force that shapes our lives. It can be external, such as changes in our environment, relationships, or circumstances, or internal, such as shifts in our beliefs, perspectives, or self-identity. Recognizing and accepting the fluid nature of life allows us to navigate change with greater resilience and adaptability.

Embracing the Unknown

Embracing change requires a willingness to venture into the unknown. It involves relinquishing our need for control and embracing the uncertainty that accompanies new experiences. By cultivating a mindset of curiosity and openness, we can approach change with a sense of adventure, eager to explore the uncharted territories that lie ahead.

Stepping Outside the Comfort Zone

Taking risks and stepping outside our comfort zones is essential for personal growth. Comfort zones, while familiar and safe, can also become stagnant and limit our potential. By challenging ourselves to try new things, face our fears, and pursue our aspirations, we expand our horizons and unlock hidden capabilities.

Cultivating Resilience

Embracing change and taking risks require resilience—the ability to bounce back from setbacks and navigate challenges. Building resilience involves developing self-belief, maintaining a positive mindset, and cultivating coping strategies to manage stress and adversity. By strengthening our resilience, we become more equipped to embrace change and thrive in the face of uncertainty.

Embracing Change as an Opportunity for Growth

Change provides fertile ground for personal growth and self-discovery. It offers us the chance to reevaluate our priorities, learn new skills, and uncover hidden talents. By reframing change as an opportunity rather than a threat, we can harness its transformative potential and cultivate a sense of empowerment.

.

Managing Fear and Uncertainty

Change can evoke fear and uncertainty, triggering anxiety and resistance. In this section, we explore strategies for managing these emotions, such as practicing self-compassion, seeking support, and reframing our perspectives. By acknowledging and addressing our fears, we can navigate change with greater ease and grace.

Celebrating Progress and Learning from Setbacks

As we embrace change and take risks, it is essential to celebrate our progress and acknowledge our achievements. We also need to embrace setbacks and learn from them, understanding that they are valuable opportunities for growth and resilience. By adopting a growth mindset, we cultivate a sense of perseverance and self-compassion in the face of challenges.

Embracing change and taking risks is a transformative endeavor that empowers us to live with greater authenticity, resilience, and joy. By embracing the unknown, stepping outside our comfort zones, and viewing change as an opportunity for growth, we unlock our full potential and navigate anxiety with courage and grace. Embrace change as a catalyst for self-discovery, and remember that with each step into the unknown, you are one step closer to lasting freedom and a life filled with fulfillment.

20

Sustaining Lasting Freedom from Anxiety

Achieving lasting freedom from anxiety is a journey that requires ongoing commitment and self-care. In this final chapter, we will explore techniques and strategies for sustaining the progress you have made and cultivating a life that continues to thrive beyond anxiety. By integrating these practices into your daily life, you can maintain a sense of well-being, resilience, and lasting freedom.

Self-Awareness and Reflection

Cultivate self-awareness by regularly reflecting on your thoughts, emotions, and behaviors. Notice any patterns or triggers that may contribute to anxiety. Take time to acknowledge your progress, celebrate your successes, and identify areas for continued growth. Self-awareness serves as a compass for maintaining lasting freedom from anxiety.

Continuous Learning and Growth

Embrace a mindset of continuous learning and personal growth. Stay curious and open to new ideas, perspectives, and strategies for managing anxiety. Seek out resources, books, courses, or workshops that can deepen your understanding of anxiety and provide tools for its effective management. Commit to a lifelong journey of personal development and growth.

Consistent Self-Care Practices

self-care as an ongoing practice. Continue engaging in activities that support your physical, mental, and emotional well-being. Regularly assess and refine your self-care routine, ensuring it aligns with your evolving needs. Treat self-care as a non-negotiable commitment to yourself and make it a priority in your daily life.

Supportive Relationships

Maintain and nurture supportive relationships in your life. Surround yourself with individuals who uplift and support you on your journey. Foster connections that are understanding, empathetic, and encourage your growth and well-being. Lean on your support system when needed and reciprocate their support as well.

Mindful Awareness

Cultivate mindful awareness as a daily practice. Stay present in each moment, noticing your thoughts, emotions, and physical sensations without judgment. Use mindfulness techniques to manage stress, reduce anxiety, and maintain a sense of clarity and calm. Regularly integrate mindfulness into your daily activities and interactions.

Flexibility and Adaptability

Embrace the reality of life's changes and uncertainties. Practice flexibility and adaptability in the face of challenges or unexpected events. Recognize that anxiety may resurface at times, but you now have the tools and resilience to navigate it effectively. Adapt your strategies as needed and approach obstacles as opportunities for growth.

Celebrating Progress

Celebrate your progress and milestones along the way. Acknowledge the steps you have taken, the challenges you have overcome, and the growth you have experienced. Give yourself credit for the resilience and courage you have shown in managing anxiety. Celebrating progress reinforces your ability to sustain lasting freedom.

Embracing a Balanced Lifestyle

Maintain a balanced lifestyle that supports your well-being. Strive for a healthy work-life balance, incorporating time for relaxation, hobbies, and meaningful connections. Avoid excessive stress or overcommitment that may trigger anxiety. Prioritize activities and commitments that align with your passions, purpose, and overall well-being.

Revisit Strategies and Techniques

Regularly revisit the strategies and techniques that have been effective in managing anxiety for you. Ensure that you continue to implement them consistently and adapt them to your changing circumstances. Stay proactive in managing anxiety, remaining open to new approaches and refining existing ones.

Remember, sustaining lasting freedom from anxiety is an ongoing journey that requires self-compassion, patience, and dedication. Embrace the process of growth and change, knowing that you have the power to live a fulfilling and anxiety-free life. Trust in your resilience and the progress you have made, and keep moving forward with confidence and determination.

Congratulations on your commitment to lasting freedom from anxiety. May your journey be filled with resilience, joy, and a sense of profound well-being.

This concludes our exploration of empowering strategies and techniques for managing anxiety, fostering resilience, and achieving lasting freedom.

21

Conclusion

Your Journey to Lasting Freedom

Congratulations on completing this transformative journey towards lasting freedom from anxiety. Throughout this book, we have explored the depths of anxiety, unraveling its grip and discovering empowering strategies to overcome its limitations. As you reach the end of this journey, remember that your path to lasting freedom is a personal and ongoing one—one that requires commitment, self-compassion, and the continuous application of the knowledge and techniques you have gained.

You have embarked on a journey of self-discovery, courageously exploring the complexities of anxiety and uncovering the power within you to transcend its hold. You have gained a deeper understanding of anxiety's nature, its causes, and the impact it has on your daily life. With this understanding, you have shifted your mindset, embracing new perspectives and empowering beliefs that allow you to navigate anxiety with resilience and strength.

Along the way, you have discovered empowering strategies and techniques for managing anxiety. You have learned to cultivate mindfulness, harness the power of your breath, and engage in practices that support your physical, mental, and emotional well-being. You have built a supportive lifestyle, nurturing relationships, setting boundaries, and prioritizing self-care. You have tapped into your passions and purpose, embracing a life aligned with your deepest desires and values. Through gratitude, self-reflection, and resilience-building, you have cultivated a mindset and environment that sustain your journey towards lasting freedom.

Remember that your journey does not end here. Lasting freedom is not a destination but a continuous process of growth, self-care, and self-discovery. As life unfolds, new challenges and opportunities will arise, and you will have the strength and tools to navigate them with grace. Embrace the lessons you have learned, celebrate your progress, and remain open to further growth and learning.

Always remember that you are not alone on this journey. Seek support from loved ones, professionals, or support groups when needed. Surround yourself with a network of understanding and compassionate individuals who uplift and support you along the way. Together, we can overcome the obstacles that anxiety presents and create a world where lasting freedom is possible for everyone.

As you step forward into the world, know that you have the power within you to thrive beyond anxiety. Trust in your resilience, embrace the practices that have served you, and remain committed to your well-being. Your journey to lasting freedom is a testament to your strength, courage, and determination. Embrace each day as an opportunity to live fully, with purpose, joy, and a deep sense of fulfillment.

May your path be filled with resilience, growth, and the unwavering belief in your ability to transcend anxiety's grip. You are capable, you are deserving, and you are on the path to lasting freedom. Embrace this newfound freedom with open arms, and may it guide you to a life of limitless possibilities.

Wishing you a future filled with lasting freedom, joy, and fulfillment.

With gratitude and support,
  Alexander Grant